PLANT BASED DIET
BUDGET MEAL PREP

The easy,healthy,quick recipes cookbook for beginners.

SHELLEY WEBSTER

TABLE OF CONTENTS

fewer animal products, you're contributing to reduced greenhouse gas emissions, water usage, and deforestation. Choosing plant-based options supports a more sustainable planet.   35

5. **Variety and Creativity:** Plant-based diets encourage culinary exploration with a wide array of fruits, vegetables, grains, legumes, nuts, and seeds. This variety can lead to exciting and diverse meals that are also budget-conscious.   35

6. **Less Food Waste:** Plant-based diets often prioritize perishable items like fruits and vegetables, reducing the likelihood of food spoilage and waste. This can lead to less frequent grocery trips and greater overall savings.   36

7. **Longevity:** Studies suggest that plant-based diets are associated with increased lifespan and improved quality of life due to their positive effects on heart health, blood pressure, and cholesterol levels.   36

8. **Educational Opportunity:** Adopting a budget-friendly plant-based diet can encourage learning about cooking techniques, nutrition, and food preparation. This knowledge can be empowering and translate to lifelong habits.   36

9. **Supports Local Agriculture:** Purchasing local, in-season plant-based foods not only supports local farmers but can also be more cost-effective compared to imported or out-of-season produce.   37

10. **Ethical Considerations:** For those

6. **Peas:** Both green peas and split peas are affordable protein sources that can be used in soups, stews, and casseroles.

7. **Quinoa:** Quinoa is a complete protein that can be used as a base for salads, bowls, and side dishes. While it's slightly more expensive than some other grains, a little goes a long way.

8. **Seitan:** Seitan, also known as wheat gluten, is a high-protein meat substitute that can be used in dishes like stir-fries, sandwiches, and sausages.

9. **Nuts and Seeds:** While nuts and seeds can be pricier, they offer protein along with healthy fats. Use them as toppings for oatmeal, yogurt, and salads, or enjoy them as a snack.

10. **Nutritional Yeast:** Nutritional yeast is a complete protein and provides a cheesy flavor to dishes. It's often used as a topping for popcorn, pasta, and roasted vegetables.

11. **Eggs:** If you include eggs in your plant-based diet, they can be an affordable and versatile protein source for meals like scrambled eggs, omelets, and frittatas.

12. **Homemade Protein Bars and Balls:** Making your own protein bars or energy balls using ingredients like oats, nut butter, and seeds can be more cost-effective than buying pre-packaged options.

13. **Plant-Based Protein Powder:** While this isn't a whole food, plant-based option, it can be cost-effective when used sparingly to supplement your protein intake.

top with fruits, nuts, and seeds.For a breakfast that is prepared,Allow it to chill in the fridge all night.   56

2. **Smoothie Bowl:** Blend frozen fruits, such as berries or bananas, with plant-based yogurt or milk.   57

3. **Avocado Toast:** Mash ripe avocado onto whole-grain toast.Sliced tomatoes, salt, pepper, and olive oil are added as garnishes. Add a touch of red pepper flakes for extra flavor.   57

4. **Chia Pudding:** Mix chia seeds with plant-based milk and sweetener.Refrigerate it for a few hours or overnight to thicken it. 57

5. **Fruit Salad:** Prepare a colorful mix of your favorite fresh fruits like berries, melon, kiwi, and oranges. Add a sprinkle of chopped nuts or a dollop of plant-based yogurt.   58

6. **Peanut Butter Banana Wrap:** Spread peanut or almond butter on a whole-grain tortilla. Place sliced bananas on top and fold the tortilla into a wrap.   58

7. **Tofu Scramble:** Crumble firm tofu and sauté with chopped vegetables like bell peppers, onions, and spinach.   58

8. **Homemade Granola:** Mix rolled oats, nuts, seeds, dried fruits, and a drizzle of maple syrup. Bake until golden brown for a crunchy homemade granola. Serve with plant-based milk or yogurt.   59

9. **Energy Balls:** Blend dates, nuts, seeds, and a bit of cocoa powder in a food processor. Roll the mixture into bite-sized

3. **Label and Date:** Always label your containers with the name of the dish and the date it was prepared. This helps you keep track of what's in your freezer and ensures you use items before they get too old.   77

4. **Portion Control:** Divide larger batches into individual or family-sized portions before freezing. This makes it easier to defrost and prevents you from having to thaw more than you need.   77

5. **Cool Down Before Freezing:** Allow hot foods to cool down before placing them in the freezer. This prevents the rise in temperature that can affect other items in the freezer.   77

6. **Use Freezer-Friendly Containers:** Choose containers designed for freezing. Glass, plastic, and freezer-safe bags work well. In order to prevent freezer burn, make sure they are airtight.   78

7. **Eliminate Air:** When using bags, press out as much air as possible before sealing to prevent freezer burn and maintain the quality of the food.   78

8. **Flash Freeze:** If you're freezing items individually, like berries, spread them out on a baking sheet before transferring to a container. This prevents them from sticking together.   78

9. **Thawing Safely:** Always thaw food in the refrigerator, not on the counter. This helps prevent bacterial growth. If you're in a rush, use the defrost setting on your microwave.   79

10. **Reheat Properly:** Reheat frozen

3. **First In, First Out**: When organizing your fridge and pantry, follow the "first in, first out" rule. Place older items at the front so they are used before newer ones.

4. **Use Leftovers Creatively**: Get creative with using leftovers. Turn them into soups, stews, sandwiches, or salads. Leftover vegetables can be used in stir-fries, omelets, or casseroles.

5. **Regrow Vegetables**: Some vegetables like green onions, lettuce, and celery can be regrown from scraps.This can help you save money and cut down on trash.

6. **Composting**: Set up a compost bin for food scraps that can't be used. This nutrient-rich compost can be used in your garden, reducing the need for store-bought fertilizers.

7. **Understand Expiry Dates**: Understand the difference between "sell by," "use by," and "best by" dates. These dates often indicate quality rather than safety. Trust your senses to determine if food is still good to eat.

8. **Portion Control**: Serve appropriate portion sizes to avoid overeating and having leftovers that might go to waste.

9. **Donate**: If you have non-perishable items that you won't use, consider donating them to local food banks or shelters.

10. **Preserve and Pickle**: Preserve excess fruits and vegetables through techniques like canning, pickling, or making jams and sauces.

major contributor to greenhouse gas emissions, deforestation, and water usage. 128

3. Culinary Creativity: Plant-based eating encourages you to explore new flavors, ingredients, and cooking methods. This can lead to greater culinary creativity and a more diverse palate. 128

4. Sustainable Eating Habits: Learning to prioritize seasonal and local produce, minimize food waste, and prepare meals at home fosters sustainable eating habits that benefit both your health and the planet. 128

5. Budget Freedom: Plant-based eating can be cost-effective, freeing up funds for other priorities in your life. With smart shopping, meal planning, and batch cooking, you can stretch your budget without compromising nutrition. 129

6. Ethical Considerations: By choosing plant-based options, you're making a compassionate choice for animals and supporting ethical food practices. 129

7. Positive Community Impact: Sharing your plant-based journey with friends and family can inspire others to make more sustainable and health-conscious choices. 129

DAILY MEAL REMARKS 130

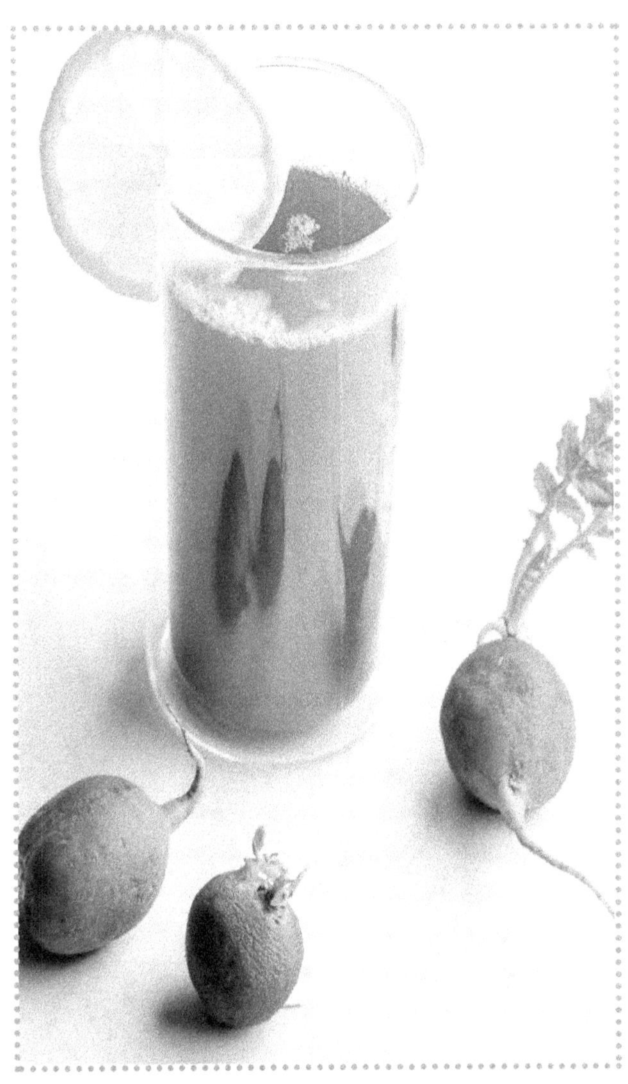

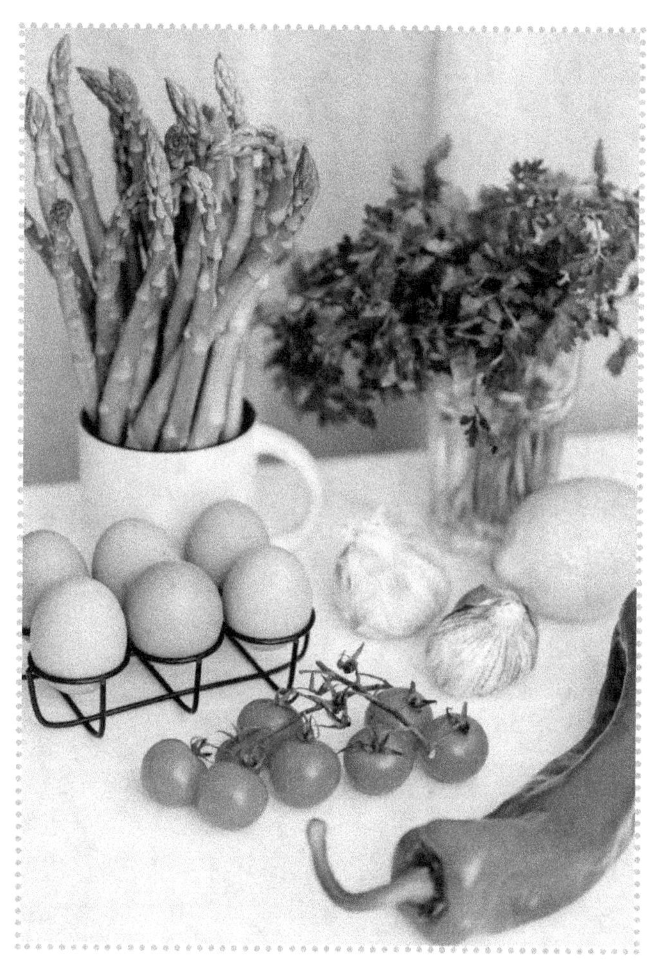

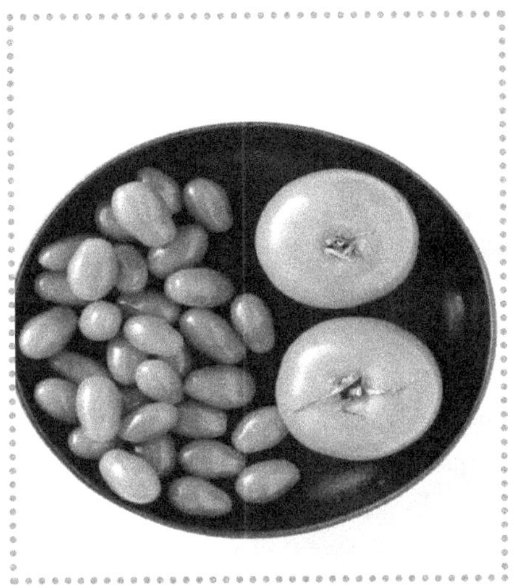

INTRODUCTION

Welcome to the world of plant-based diet budget meal prep! In this guide, we'll explore how to create delicious, nutritious, and wallet-friendly meals centered around plant-based ingredients. Whether you're a seasoned plant-based eater or just starting to incorporate more plants into your diet, we'll provide you with practical tips, affordable ingredient ideas, and efficient meal prep strategies to help you embrace a healthier lifestyle without breaking the bank. Let's embark on a journey of flavorful and budget-conscious plant.

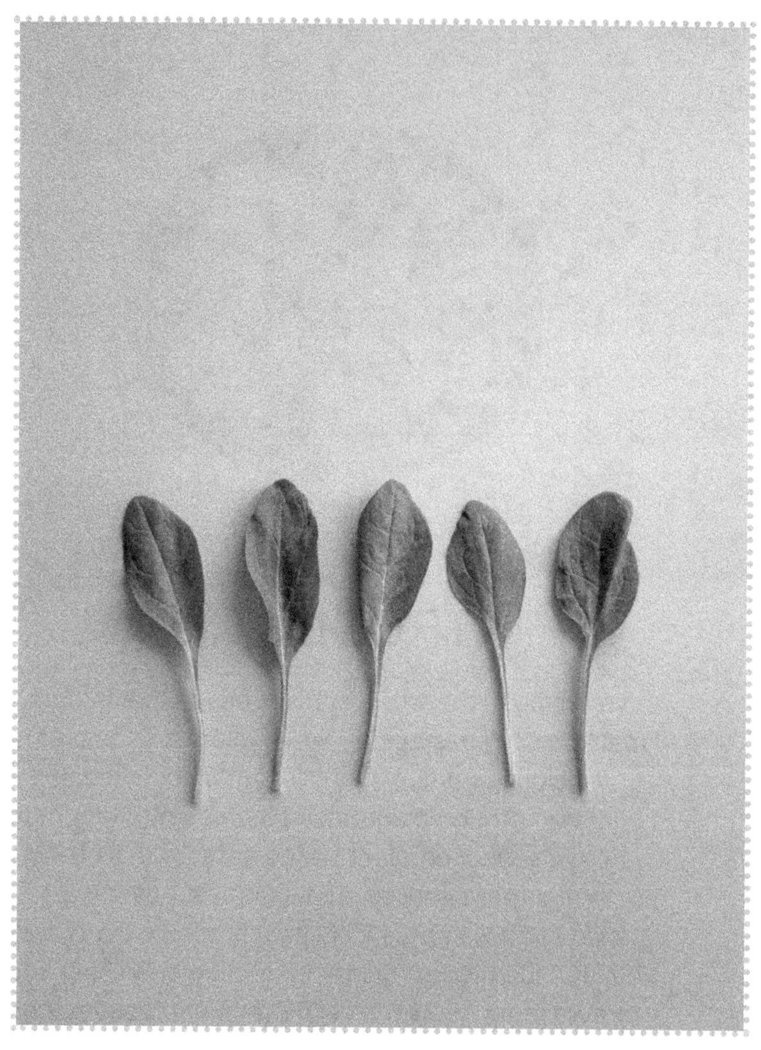

CHAPTER ONE

A PLANT-BASED DIET'S BENEFITS FOR A BUDGET

1. **Cost Savings:** Plant-based diets often rely on affordable staples like beans, lentils, grains, and seasonal produce, making them more budget-friendly compared to animal-based diets that can be higher in cost.

2. **Improved Health:** Plant-based diets are associated with lower risks of chronic diseases such as heart disease, diabetes, and certain cancers. By prioritizing whole plant foods, you can potentially reduce healthcare costs in the long run.

3. **Weight Management:** Plant-based diets tend to be lower in calories and saturated fats, making them conducive to weight loss and maintenance without the need for expensive diet programs or supplements.

4. **Environmental Impact:** By consuming fewer animal products, you're contributing to reduced greenhouse gas emissions, water usage, and deforestation. Choosing plant-based options supports a more sustainable planet.

5. **Variety and Creativity:** Plant-based diets encourage culinary exploration with a wide array of fruits, vegetables, grains, legumes, nuts, and seeds. This variety can lead to exciting and diverse meals that are also budget-conscious.

6. **Less Food Waste:** Plant-based diets often prioritize perishable items like fruits and vegetables, reducing the likelihood of food spoilage and waste. This can lead to less frequent grocery trips and greater overall savings.

7. **Longevity:** Studies suggest that plant-based diets are associated with increased lifespan and improved quality of life due to their positive effects on heart health, blood pressure, and cholesterol levels.

8. **Educational Opportunity:** Adopting a budget-friendly plant-based diet can encourage learning about cooking techniques, nutrition, and food preparation. This knowledge can be empowering and translate to lifelong habits.

9. **Supports Local Agriculture:** Purchasing local, in-season plant-based foods not only supports local farmers but can also be more cost-effective compared to imported or out-of-season produce.

10. **Ethical Considerations:** For those concerned about animal welfare, a plant-based diet aligns with ethical values, promoting compassion for animals without compromising financial constraints.

Remember, a plant-based diet doesn't have to be an all-or-nothing commitment. Incorporating more plant-based meals into your routine, even on a budget, can still provide substantial benefits for both your health and your finances.

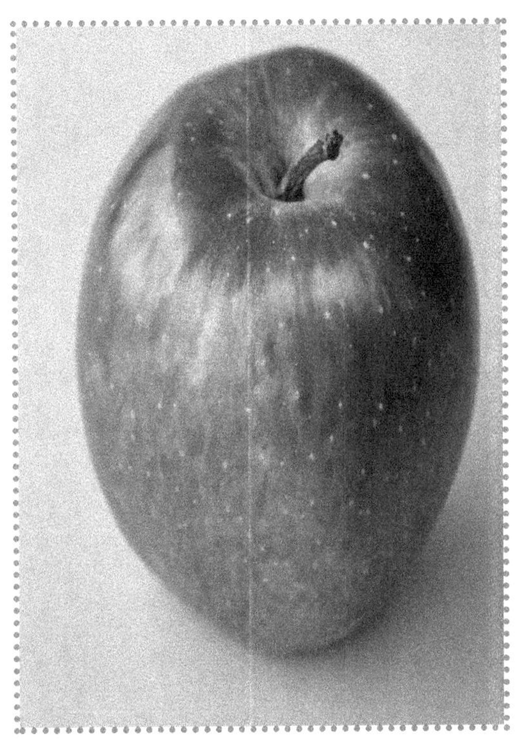

CHAPTER TWO

ESSENTIAL PANTRY STAPLES

Building a well-stocked pantry is essential for successful plant-based meal prep on a budget. Here are some must-have pantry staples that will form the foundation of your plant-based cooking:

1. **Grains:** Quinoa, brown rice, whole wheat pasta, oats, couscous, and bulgur are versatile and provide essential carbohydrates.

2. **Legumes:** Stock up on dried or canned beans (black beans, chickpeas, lentils, kidney beans) for protein and fiber-rich options that can be used in various dishes.

3. **Canned Tomatoes:** Whole, diced, or crushed tomatoes serve as a base for sauces, stews, and soups.

4. **Nuts and Seeds:** Almonds, walnuts, chia seeds, flaxseeds, and sunflower seeds are great sources of healthy fats and added texture to dishes.

5. **Nut Butters:** Peanut butter, almond butter, or tahini are protein-packed and can be used in both sweet and savory recipes.

6. **Plant-Based Milk:** Options like almond, soy, oat, or coconut milk can be used in cooking, baking, and as a dairy milk substitute.

7. **Flour:** Whole wheat flour, almond flour, and all-purpose flour are useful for baking and thickening sauces.

8. **Spices and Herbs:** Basics like garlic powder, onion powder, cumin, paprika, oregano, and basil add flavor to your dishes.

9. **Condiments and Sauces:** Soy sauce, vinegar (balsamic, apple cider, rice), hot sauce, and mustard can enhance the taste of your meals.

10. **Oils:** Olive oil, coconut oil, and sesame oil are essential for cooking and flavoring.

11. **Whole-Grain Pasta:** Opt for whole wheat or legume-based pasta for added nutrients and fiber.

12. **Dried Fruits:** Raisins, apricots, cranberries, and dates add natural sweetness to recipes.

13. **Sweeteners:** Agave syrup, maple syrup, and coconut sugar are plant-based alternatives to refined sugars.

14. **Canned or Jarred Sauces:** Salsa, marinara sauce, and curry paste can simplify meal prep.

15. **Veggies and Fruits** (Canned or Frozen):** Items like corn, peas, and spinach can be convenient additions when fresh produce isn't available.

16. **Whole-Grain Cereals:** Look for low-sugar options made from oats, quinoa, or bran.

17. **Dried Herbs:** Rosemary, thyme, sage, and parsley can elevate the flavor of your dishes.

18. **Rice and Noodles:** Brown rice noodles, rice paper wraps, and rice noodles are versatile for creating stir-fries and wraps.

19. **Vegetable Broth:** A versatile base for soups, stews, and risottos.

Plant-Based Protein: Textured vegetable protein (TVP), tempeh, and tofu are excellent protein sources.

Having these essential pantry staples on hand will enable you to create a wide variety of plant-based meals without constantly needing to run to the store. By combining these ingredients with fresh produce, you'll have the tools to whip up delicious and nutritious dishes while sticking to your budget.

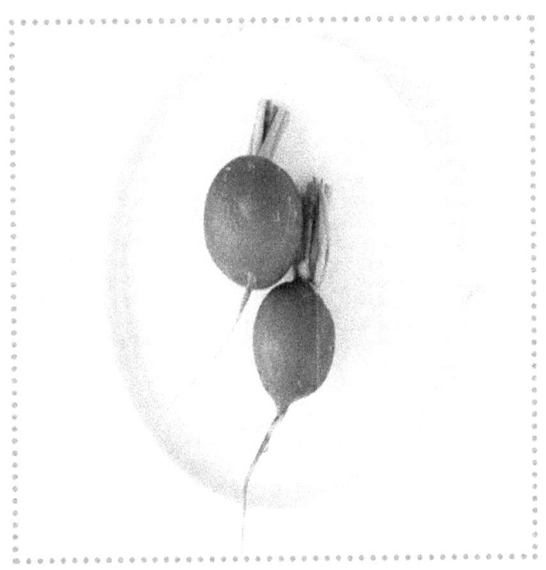

CHAPTER THREE

COST EFFECTIVE PROTEIN SOURCES

When following a plant-based diet on a budget, it's important to choose cost-effective protein sources that provide the necessary nutrients without straining your wallet. Here are some affordable plant-based protein options to consider:

1. **Beans and Legumes:** Beans like black beans, kidney beans, pinto beans, and lentils are protein powerhouses and are incredibly budget-friendly. They can be included in salads, vegetarian burgers made from scratch, and even soups and stews.

2. **Chickpeas:** Versatile and rich in protein, chickpeas can be roasted for snacking, blended into hummus, or added to curries and salads.

3. **Tofu:** Tofu is an excellent source of protein and can be marinated, grilled, stir-fried, or blended into smoothies. It's often one of the more affordable protein options in the grocery store.

4. **Tempeh:** Tempeh is a fermented soy product that offers a hearty texture and a good amount of protein. It absorbs flavors well and can be used in sandwiches, stir-fries, and salads.

5. **Textured Vegetable Protein (TVP):** TVP is a versatile and economical option. It's often used as a meat substitute in recipes like chili, tacos, and spaghetti sauce.

6. **Peas:** Both green peas and split peas are affordable protein sources that can be used in soups, stews, and casseroles.

7. **Quinoa:** Quinoa is a complete protein that can be used as a base for salads, bowls, and side dishes. While it's slightly more expensive than some other grains, a little goes a long way.

8. **Seitan:** Seitan, also known as wheat gluten, is a high-protein meat substitute that can be used in dishes like stir-fries, sandwiches, and sausages.

9. **Nuts and Seeds:** While nuts and seeds can be pricier, they offer protein along with healthy fats. Use them as toppings for oatmeal, yogurt, and salads, or enjoy them as a snack.

10. **Nutritional Yeast:** Nutritional yeast is a complete protein and provides a cheesy flavor to dishes. It's often used as a topping for popcorn, pasta, and roasted vegetables.

11. **Eggs:** If you include eggs in your plant-based diet, they can be an affordable and versatile protein source for meals like scrambled eggs, omelets, and frittatas.

12. **Homemade Protein Bars and Balls:** Making your own protein bars or energy balls using ingredients like oats, nut butter, and seeds can be more cost-effective than buying pre-packaged options.

13. **Plant-Based Protein Powder:**
While this isn't a whole food, plant-based option, it can be cost-effective when used sparingly to supplement your protein intake.

Remember that incorporating a variety of these protein sources into your meals can help you meet your protein needs while staying within your budget. Also, purchasing items in bulk and taking advantage of sales and discounts can further reduce costs. With a little creativity and planning, you can enjoy ample protein on a plant-based diet without overspending.

Embracing seasonal and local produce not only enhances the flavor of your meals but also saves you money. When you choose fruits and vegetables that are in season, they tend to be at their peak flavor and nutritional value. Additionally, local produce requires less transportation, reducing carbon emissions and supporting your community's economy. To maximize savings, consider shopping at farmers' markets or joining a community-supported agriculture (CSA) program. Planning your meals around what's in season can inspire creativity in the kitchen and lead to a more sustainable and budget-friendly lifestyle.

CHAPTER FOUR

Meal Planning Strategies for Budget Success

Meal planning is a powerful strategy to achieve budget success without compromising on nutrition or taste. Here are some effective tips:

1. **Plan Ahead:** Set aside time each week to plan your meals. Consider your schedule, available ingredients, and dietary preferences.

2. **Create a Menu:** Design a menu for the week based on the meals you'll prepare. Include breakfast, lunch, dinner, and snacks.

3. **Use What You Have:** Check your pantry, fridge, and freezer for ingredients you already have. Incorporate them into your plan to minimize waste.

4. **Shop with a List:** Make a detailed shopping list based on your menu. Stick to the list to avoid impulse purchases that can strain your budget.

5. **Buy in Bulk:** Staples like rice, pasta, and beans are often cheaper in bulk. Buy larger quantities when on sale, and portion them for different meals.

6. **Embrace Frozen and Canned Foods:** These options are often more affordable and have a longer shelf life. Frozen fruits, vegetables, and canned goods can be used in a variety of dishes.

7. **Cook in Batches:** Prepare larger quantities of meals and freeze individual portions. This prevents the urge to order takeout on busy nights.

8. **Repurpose Leftovers:** Get creative with leftovers. Turn roasted chicken into sandwiches or add cooked vegetables to a frittata.

9. **Focus on Versatile Ingredients:** Choose ingredients that can be used in multiple dishes. For example, a roast chicken can be part of a main dish one night and a salad the next.

10. **Minimize Meat Consumption:** Meat can be expensive. Opt for plant-based protein sources like legumes, tofu, and eggs to reduce costs.

11. **Plan for Flexible Meals:** Include a couple of "flex" meals that can be easily adjusted based on what's available or on sale.

12. **Use Apps and Tools:** There are meal planning apps that help you organize recipes, generate shopping lists, and track your budget.

13. **Bulk Cooking:** Cook large portions of staple foods like rice or quinoa to use in multiple meals throughout the week.

14. **Limit Eating Out:** Reserve eating out for special occasions to save money. Homemade meals are more cost-effective.

15. **Monitor Sales and Discounts:** Keep an eye on sales, coupons, and discounts at your local grocery store. Plan meals around discounted items.

By adopting these meal planning strategies, you can take control of your budget while enjoying nutritious and flavorful meals.

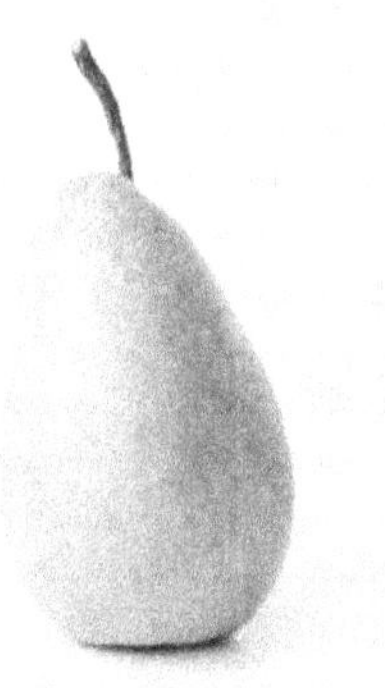

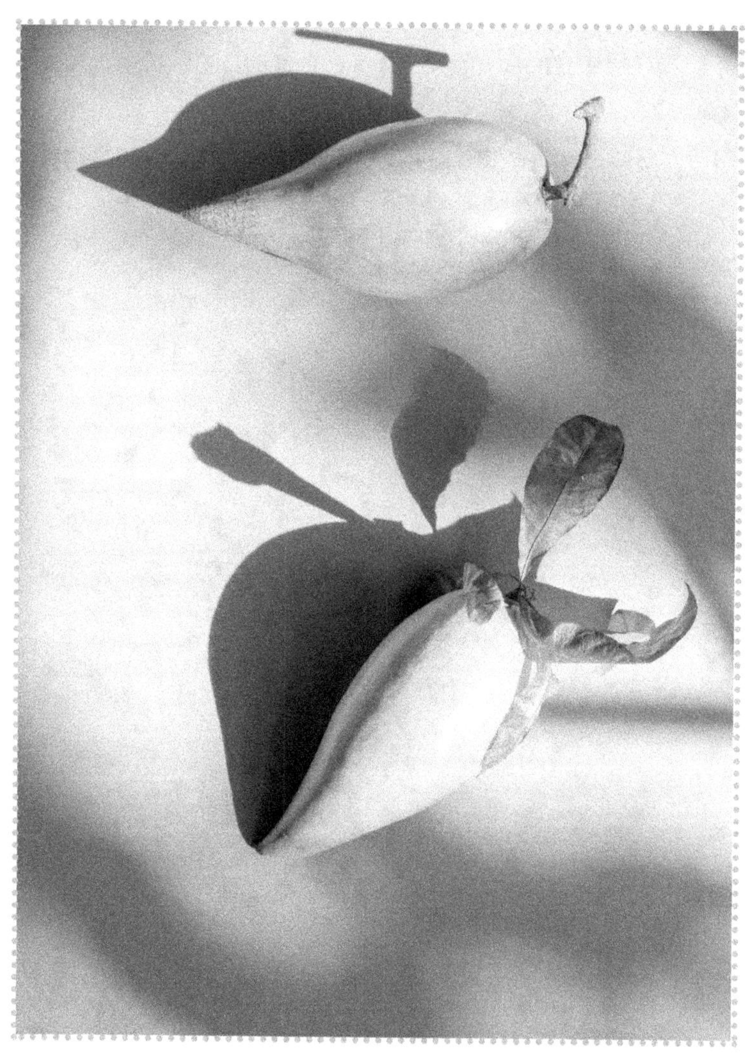

CHAPTER FIVE

Quick and Easy Breakfast Ideas

Certainly! Here are some quick and easy plant-based breakfast ideas that are both nutritious and delicious:

1. **Overnight Oats:** Mix rolled oats with your choice of plant-based milk, add sweeteners like maple syrup or honey, and top with fruits, nuts, and seeds.For a breakfast that is prepared,Allow it to chill in the fridge all night.

2. **Smoothie Bowl:** Blend frozen fruits, such as berries or bananas, with plant-based yogurt or milk.

Place the smoothie in a bowl and top with chia seeds, granola, and sliced fruit.

3. **Avocado Toast:** Mash ripe avocado onto whole-grain toast.Sliced tomatoes, salt, pepper, and olive oil are added as garnishes. Add a touch of red pepper flakes for extra flavor.

4. **Chia Pudding:** Mix chia seeds with plant-based milk and sweetener.Refrigerate it for a few hours or overnight to thicken it.

Top with fresh fruits and nuts before serving.

5. **Fruit Salad:** Prepare a colorful mix
of your favorite fresh fruits like berries,
melon, kiwi, and oranges. Add a sprinkle
of chopped nuts or a dollop of
plant-based yogurt.

6. **Peanut Butter Banana Wrap:**
Spread peanut or almond butter on a
whole-grain tortilla. Place sliced
bananas on top and fold the tortilla into
a wrap.

7. **Tofu Scramble:** Crumble firm tofu
and sauté with chopped vegetables like
bell peppers, onions, and spinach.
For a tasty scramble, season with turmeric, cumin,
and nutritional yeast.

8. **Homemade Granola:** Mix rolled oats, nuts, seeds, dried fruits, and a drizzle of maple syrup. Bake until golden brown for a crunchy homemade granola. Serve with plant-based milk or yogurt.

9. **Energy Balls:** Blend dates, nuts, seeds, and a bit of cocoa powder in a food processor. Roll the mixture into bite-sized balls for a quick grab-and-go option.

10. **Whole-Grain Cereal:** Opt for whole-grain cereal with plant-based milk. Add sliced fruits, nuts, and a sprinkle of cinnamon for extra flavor.

11. **Vegan Pancakes:** Make pancakes using a plant-based milk and flaxseed meal as an egg substitute. Top with berries, sliced bananas, or a drizzle of pure maple syrup.

12. **Breakfast Burrito:** Fill a whole-grain tortilla with black beans, sautéed veggies, salsa, and a sprinkle of nutritional yeast for a savory breakfast burrito.

13. **Rice Cake Delight:** Top rice cakes with almond or peanut butter, sliced fruits, and a sprinkle of hemp seeds for added protein.

14. **Fruit and Nut Parfait:** Layer plant-based yogurt with chopped fruits, nuts, and a touch of honey or agave for a refreshing and satisfying parfait.

15. **Leftover Dinner Remix:** Sometimes leftovers from a plant-based dinner can make a quick and nutritious breakfast. Reheat veggie stir-fries or bean-based dishes for a convenient morning meal.

These plant-based breakfast ideas are not only quick and easy to prepare but also provide a range of nutrients to kick-start your day.

CHAPTER SIX

Budget-Friendly Lunch Recipes

Absolutely, here are a few budget-friendly plant-based lunch recipes that you can easily prepare:

1. Chickpea Salad Wraps:

- Drain and rinse a can of chickpeas.
- Mash them slightly with a fork and mix with diced veggies (cucumber, bell pepper, red onion).
- Add chopped fresh herbs (parsley, cilantro), a squeeze of lemon juice, salt, pepper, and a drizzle of olive oil.
- Spoon the mixture onto whole wheat tortillas or lettuce leaves, wrap, and enjoy.

2. Lentil and Vegetable Stir-Fry:

- Cook lentils until tender, then drain.
- In a pan, stir-fry chopped mixed vegetables (carrots, broccoli, bell peppers) with garlic and ginger.

- Add cooked lentils and a simple stir-fry sauce
made from soy sauce, a touch of sweetener, and a
splash of vegetable broth.
- Serve over brown rice or quinoa.

3. Hummus Veggie Bowl:

- Spread hummus on the base of a bowl.
- Add cooked quinoa or couscous, and top with a
variety of chopped veggies (tomatoes, cucumbers,
bell peppers, carrots).
- Sprinkle with seeds (sunflower, pumpkin) and a
drizzle of olive oil or lemon-tahini dressing.

4. Black Bean Quesadillas:

- Mash black beans with spices (cumin, chili
powder) and a touch of salsa.
- Spread the mixture on a tortilla, top with shredded
vegan cheese and another tortilla.
- Cook on a non-stick pan until the tortillas are
crispy and the cheese is melted.
- Slice into wedges and serve with salsa or
guacamole.

5. Vegetable and Rice Bowl:

- Sauté a mix of your favorite vegetables (zucchini,
bell peppers, onions) with a bit of soy sauce and
garlic.

- Serve over cooked brown rice, and optionally sprinkle with sesame seeds or crushed peanuts.

6. Pasta with Marinara and Veggies:

- Cook whole-grain pasta according to package instructions.
- Heat up store-bought or homemade marinara sauce.
- Add sautéed veggies (spinach, mushrooms, zucchini) and mix with the cooked pasta.
- Garnish with fresh basil and a sprinkle of nutritional yeast.

7. DIY Salad Bar:

- Prepare a variety of salad greens, chopped veggies, beans, and grains.
- Create your own salad with a mix of ingredients and top with a simple vinaigrette made from olive oil, vinegar, mustard, and seasoning.

These lunch recipes are not only budget-friendly but also nutritious and satisfying. Feel free to customize them based on your taste preferences

and the ingredients you have on hand. Happy cooking!

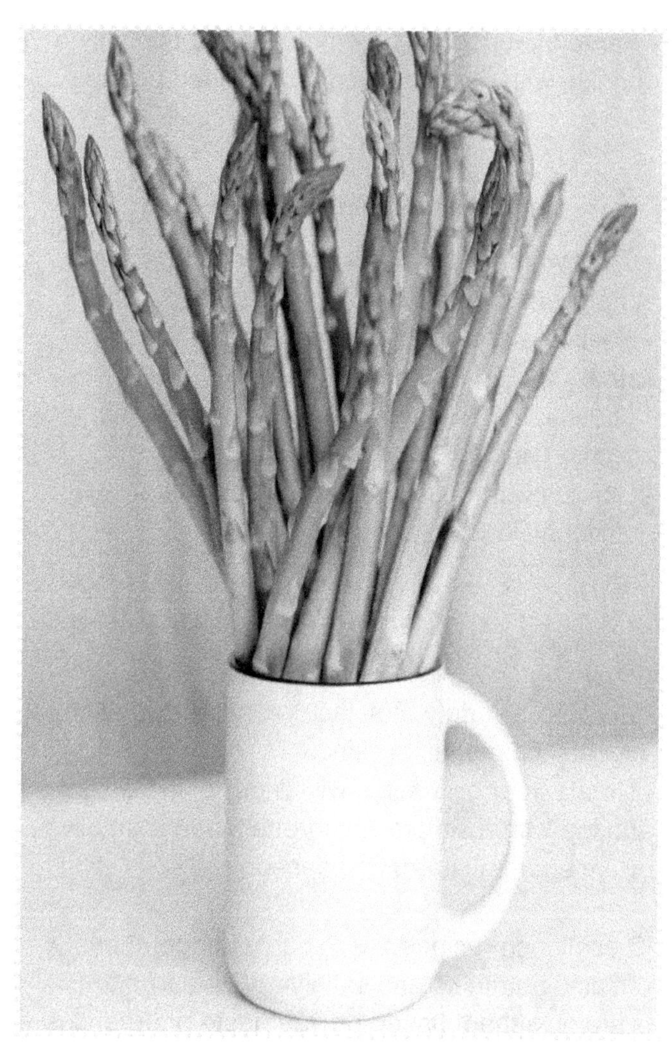

CHAPTER SEVEN

Nutrient-Packed Dinners on a Budget

Certainly! Here are some nutrient-packed dinner ideas that are both budget-friendly and plant-based:

1. Lentil and Vegetable Stew:

- Sauté onions, carrots, and celery in a pot until softened.
- Add red or green lentils and vegetable broth, then simmer until lentils are cooked.
- Add chopped tomatoes, spinach, and your favorite spices.
- Serve with whole-grain bread or rice for a hearty and filling stew.

2. Vegetable Stir-Fry with Tofu:

- Sauté tofu cubes until golden brown, then set aside.
- In the same pan, stir-fry a mix of vegetables (broccoli, bell peppers, snap peas) with garlic and ginger.

- Add back the tofu and a simple stir-fry sauce made from soy sauce, sesame oil, and a touch of sweetener.
- Serve over brown rice or noodles.

3. Quinoa and Black Bean Bowl:

- Cook quinoa and set aside.
- Sauté black beans with spices (cumin, paprika) and garlic.
- Assemble bowls with quinoa, beans, diced tomatoes, corn, avocado, and a drizzle of lime juice.
- Top with fresh cilantro and a dollop of salsa.

4. Veggie and Chickpea Curry:

- Sauté onions, garlic, and ginger in a pot until fragrant.
- Add your favorite curry spices (turmeric, cumin, coriander), then stir in diced vegetables (potatoes, cauliflower, carrots).
- Pour in canned chickpeas and coconut milk, and simmer until vegetables are tender.
- Serve over cooked brown rice or whole wheat naan.

5. One-Pot Pasta Primavera:

- In a large pot, sauté diced veggies (zucchini, bell peppers, cherry tomatoes) until slightly softened.
- Add whole wheat pasta, vegetable broth, and water, and simmer until the pasta is cooked and the liquid is absorbed.
- Stir in fresh herbs (basil, parsley) and a squeeze of lemon juice before serving.

6. Stuffed Bell Peppers:

- Cut the tops off bell peppers and remove seeds.
- Mix cooked quinoa with black beans, corn, diced tomatoes, and spices.
- Stuff the mixture into the peppers and bake until the peppers are tender.
- Top with vegan cheese and broil until melted.

7. Roasted Vegetable and Hummus Bowl:

- Roast a variety of vegetables (sweet potatoes, cauliflower, Brussels sprouts) with olive oil and spices.
- Serve the roasted veggies over a bed of quinoa or brown rice.
- Add dollops of hummus, a sprinkle of nuts or seeds, and a drizzle of balsamic glaze.

These nutrient-packed dinner ideas are not only delicious and satisfying but also easy on the wallet. Customize them based on your preferences and available ingredients to create budget-friendly meals that nourish your body.

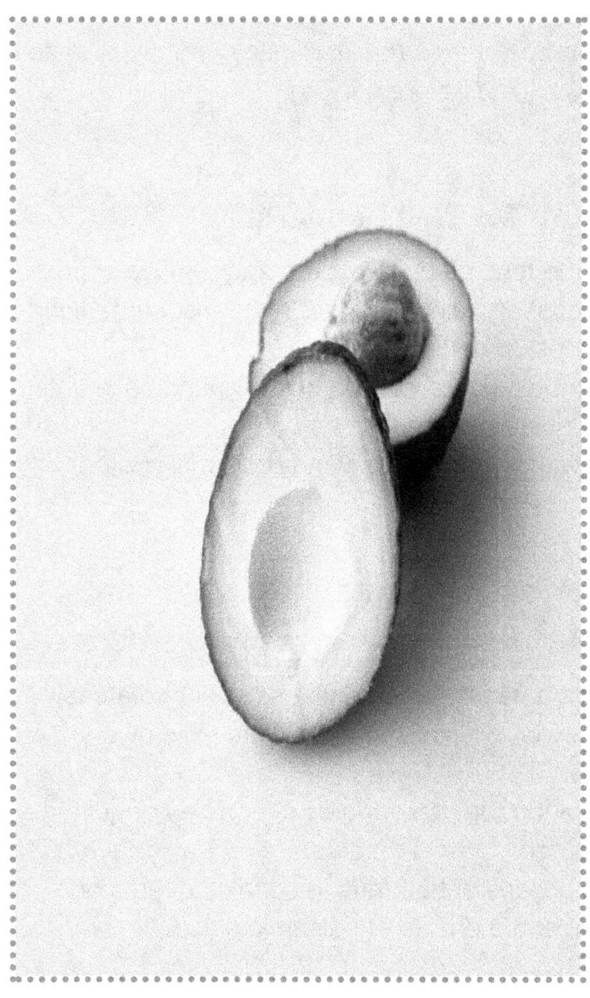

CHAPTER EIGHT

Snacking Smart: Affordable

Absolutely, here are some tips and affordable plant-based snack ideas for snacking smart:

Tips for Smart Snacking on a Budget:

1. **Plan Ahead:** Set aside time to plan your snacks for the week. This will help you avoid impulse purchases and opt for budget-friendly options.

2. **Buy in Bulk:** Purchase nuts, seeds, dried fruits, and whole grains in bulk. Long-term cost-effectiveness can be achieved by purchasing greater volumes.

3. **Prepare Snacks at Home:** Making your own snacks, like energy bars, trail mix, or popcorn, can save money compared to pre-packaged options.

4. **Choose Whole Foods:** Opt for whole fruits, vegetables, and minimally processed foods. These are often more affordable and offer better nutritional value.

5. **Portion Control:** Divide bulk snacks into smaller portions to avoid overeating and stretching your budget.

CHAPTER NINE

Affordable Plant-Based Snack Ideas:

1. **Popcorn:** Air-popped popcorn is a budget-friendly and satisfying snack. Sprinkle with nutritional yeast or your favorite seasoning.

2. **Trail Mix:** Create your own trail mix using nuts, seeds, dried fruits, and a touch of dark chocolate for a sweet treat.

3. **Fresh Fruit:** Apples, bananas, oranges, and other in-season fruits are convenient and economical snacks.

4. **Carrot Sticks with Hummus:**
Carrot sticks paired with homemade or store-bought hummus offer a balanced and nutritious snack.

5. **Rice Cakes with Nut Butter:**
Spread natural nut butter (like peanut or almond) on whole-grain rice cakes for a satisfying combination of protein and carbs.

6. **Oatmeal Cups:** Make a batch of simple oatmeal cups with oats, mashed bananas, and your choice of add-ins (nuts, dried fruits, seeds).

7. **Frozen Grapes:** Freeze grapes for a refreshing and sweet snack during warmer months.

8. **Veggie Sticks with Guacamole:**
Sliced cucumbers, bell peppers, and
cherry tomatoes with guacamole provide
vitamins, fiber, and healthy fats.

9. **Rice Crackers with Salsa:** Pair
whole-grain rice crackers with a zesty
salsa for a crunchy and flavorful snack.

10. **Homemade Energy Balls:** Create
energy balls using oats, nut butter,
dates, and your choice of mix-ins like
chocolate chips or shredded coconut.

11. **DIY Smoothie:** Blend frozen
fruits, plant-based milk, and a handful of
spinach or kale for a budget-friendly
nutrient boost.

12. **Roasted Chickpeas:** Roast canned chickpeas with your favorite spices for a crunchy and protein-packed snack.

13. **Yogurt Parfait:** Layer dairy-free yogurt with granola and fresh berries for a satisfying and visually appealing snack.

14. **Apple Slices with Peanut Butter:** Dip apple slices into peanut butter for a classic and wholesome combination.

15. **Crispy Chickpea Snack:** Toss cooked chickpeas with olive oil and spices, then roast until crispy for a savory and crunchy snack.

These snack ideas are not only affordable but also nutritious, making it easier to maintain a healthy plant-based lifestyle while staying within your budget.

CHAPTER TEN

Batch Cooking and Freezing Tips

Batch cooking and freezing are fantastic strategies for saving time, reducing meal prep stress, and minimizing food waste.Here are some pointers for maximizing these methods:

1. **Plan Your Meals:** Start by selecting recipes that freeze well and are suitable for reheating. Consider dishes like stews, soups, casseroles, and sauces.

2. **Choose Appropriate Ingredients:**
Opt for ingredients that hold up well in
the freezer. Foods with high water
content (like lettuce) may not freeze as
successfully.

3. **Label and Date:** Always label your
containers with the name of the dish and
the date it was prepared. This helps you
keep track of what's in your freezer and
ensures you use items before they get
too old.

4. **Portion Control:** Divide larger
batches into individual or family-sized
portions before freezing. This makes it
easier to defrost and prevents you from
having to thaw more than you need.

5. **Cool Down Before Freezing:** Allow hot foods to cool down before placing them in the freezer. This prevents the rise in temperature that can affect other items in the freezer.

6. **Use Freezer-Friendly Containers:** Choose containers designed for freezing. Glass, plastic, and freezer-safe bags work well. In order to prevent freezer burn, make sure they are airtight.

7. **Eliminate Air:** When using bags, press out as much air as possible before sealing to prevent freezer burn and maintain the quality of the food.

8. **Flash Freeze:** If you're freezing items individually, like berries, spread them out on a baking sheet before transferring to a container. This prevents them from sticking together.

9. **Thawing Safely:** Always thaw food in the refrigerator, not on the counter. This helps prevent bacterial growth. If you're in a rush, use the defrost setting on your microwave.

10. **Reheat Properly:** Reheat frozen meals in the microwave or oven, ensuring they reach a safe internal temperature. Stirring and flipping during reheating helps distribute heat evenly.

11. **Rotate Stock:** To prevent forgotten items, use the "first in, first out" rule.Move older things to the front of the freezer and place recently frozen items at the back.

12. **Keep an Inventory:** Maintain a list of what's in your freezer to easily track what you have on hand. This prevents overbuying or missing out on items.

13. **Freezing Times:** Different dishes have varying freezer life. Generally, cooked meats can be frozen for 2-6 months, soups and stews for 2-3 months, and baked goods for 1-2 months.

14. **Texture Consideration:** Some foods may have slight changes in texture after freezing. Research which dishes freeze best to manage your expectations.

Remember that not all foods freeze well, so it's a good idea to experiment and discover what works best for your preferences. Batch cooking and freezing can truly be game-changers for meal planning and preparation.

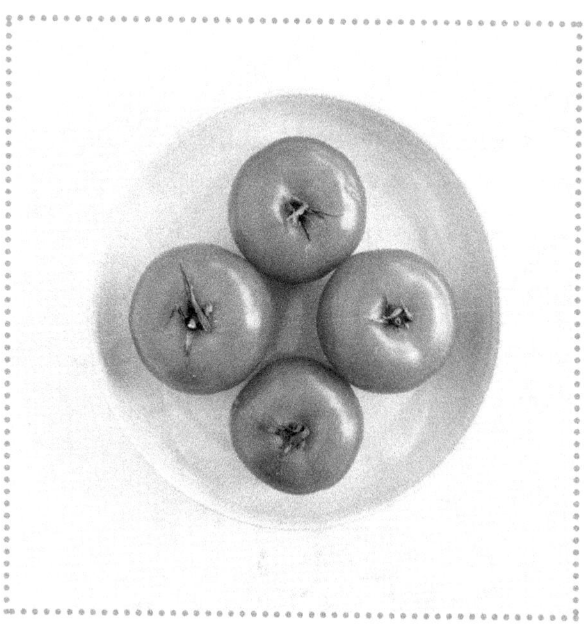

CHAPTER ELEVEN

Thrifty Tips for Reducing food waste

Certainly! Here are some thrifty tips for reducing food waste:

1. **Plan Meals**: Plan your meals for the week and create a shopping list accordingly. This helps you buy only what you need, reducing the chance of food going to waste.

2. **Proper Storage**: Store perishables like fruits, vegetables, and dairy products properly to extend their freshness. Use airtight containers and consider using the freezer for items that you won't use immediately.

3. **First In, First Out**: When organizing your fridge and pantry, follow the "first in, first out" rule. Place older items at the front so they are used before newer ones.

4. **Use Leftovers Creatively**: Get creative with using leftovers. Turn them into soups, stews, sandwiches, or salads. Leftover vegetables can be used in stir-fries, omelets, or casseroles.

5. **Regrow Vegetables**: Some vegetables like green onions, lettuce, and celery can be regrown from scraps.This can help you save money and cut down on trash.

6. **Composting**: Set up a compost bin for food scraps that can't be used. This nutrient-rich compost can be used in your garden, reducing the need for store-bought fertilizers.

7. **Understand Expiry Dates**: Understand the difference between "sell by," "use by," and "best by" dates. These dates often indicate quality rather than safety. Trust your senses to determine if food is still good to eat.

8. **Portion Control**: Serve appropriate portion sizes to avoid overeating and having leftovers that might go to waste.

9. **Donate**: If you have non-perishable items that you won't use, consider donating them to local food banks or shelters.

10. **Preserve and Pickle**: Preserve excess fruits and vegetables through techniques like canning, pickling, or making jams and sauces.

11. **Bulk Buying**: Purchase items in bulk only if you're sure you'll use them before they expire. It's only a good deal if you can consume it all.

12. **Use Every Bit**: Get creative with using the often-discarded parts of vegetables, like using broccoli stems in dishes or making stock from leftover bones.

13. **Rotate Pantry Items**: When restocking your pantry, move older items to the front and place newer items at the back. This helps ensure everything gets used before it expires.

14. **DIY Snacks**: Make your own snacks at home. This allows you to control portion sizes and avoid pre-packaged snacks that might go stale.

15. **Educate Family Members**: Teach your family about the importance of reducing food waste so everyone is on board with your efforts.

Remember, even small changes in your habits can add up to significant reductions in food waste and your grocery expenses.

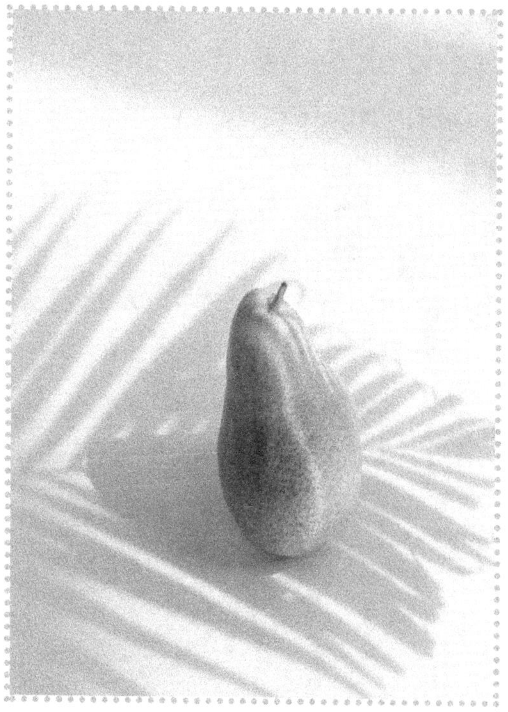

CHAPTER TWELVE

Creating a Budget-Friendly Shopping List

Creating a budget-friendly shopping list involves careful planning and prioritization. Here's how to do it:

1. **Plan Meals Ahead**: Plan your meals for the week before making the shopping list. This ensures you only buy items you'll actually use.

2. **Check Your Pantry**: Take stock of what you already have at home. This prevents you from buying items you don't need and helps you build meals around existing ingredients.

3. **Stick to Basics**: Focus on staple items like grains, proteins, and vegetables. These versatile ingredients form the foundation of many meals.

4. **Set a Budget**: Determine how much you're willing to spend on groceries for the week and stick to it. This helps avoid overspending.

5. **Buy in Bulk**: For items with a longer shelf life, consider buying in bulk. This can be cost-effective over time, but only if you'll use the items before they expire.

6. **Compare Prices**: Look for sales,
discounts, and compare prices across
different brands. Sometimes store
brands are just as good as name brands
and cost less.

7. **Opt for Seasonal Produce**:
Seasonal fruits and vegetables are often
cheaper and fresher. Incorporate these
into your meals.

8. **Avoid Pre-Packaged Foods**:
Pre-packaged or convenience foods
tend to cost more. Buy whole
ingredients and prepare meals at home.

9. **Limit Impulse Buys**: Stick to your
shopping list to avoid picking up
unnecessary items on a whim.

10. **Consider Frozen and Canned Foods**: These can be more affordable alternatives to fresh produce and are often just as nutritious.

11. **Choose Versatile Ingredients**: Opt for ingredients that can be used in multiple dishes. For example, a bag of rice or pasta can be the base for several meals.

12. **Limit Meat Purchases**: Meat can be expensive. Reduce meat consumption or choose less expensive cuts to save money.

13. **Shop at Discount Stores**: Consider shopping at discount grocery stores or farmers' markets for potentially lower prices.

14. **Avoid Shopping When Hungry**:
Shopping on an empty stomach can
lead to impulse purchases of snacks or
items not on your list.

15. **Use Coupons and Apps**: Look for
coupons or use money-saving apps that
offer discounts on grocery items.

16. **DIY Snacks and Staples**: Make
your own snacks and staples like
granola bars, salad dressings, and
sauces. It's often cheaper than buying
pre-made versions.

17. **Limit Specialty Items**: While it's
nice to try new things, specialty items
can be expensive. Save them for special
occasions.

18. **Be Mindful of Portion Sizes**:
Avoid buying more than you can
consume before it goes bad. Smaller
portions can save money in the long
run.

Remember, the key to a budget-friendly shopping
list is to plan ahead, prioritize necessities, and
make conscious choices to maximize your money's
value.

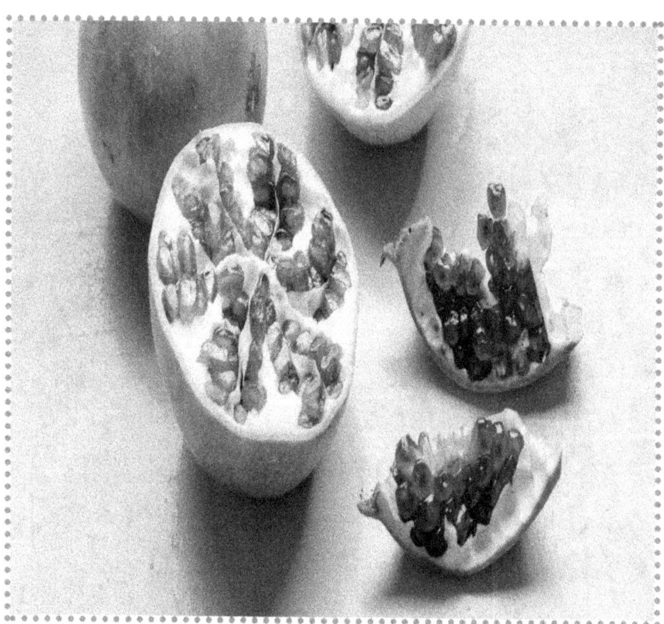

CHAPTER THIRTEEN

Cooking Tools and Equipment for Efficient Meal Prep

Efficient meal prep can be made easier with the right cooking tools and equipment. Here's a list of items that can help you streamline your cooking process:

1. **Chef's Knife**: A good quality chef's knife is essential for chopping, slicing, and dicing ingredients quickly and accurately.

2. **Cutting Board**: Invest in a sturdy cutting board to protect your countertops and provide a safe surface for chopping.

3. **Food Processor**: A food processor can chop, blend, and puree ingredients in seconds, saving you time on prep work.

4. **Blender**: A blender is great for making smoothies, soups, sauces, and even pancake batter.

5. **Mixing Bowls**: Have a set of various-sized mixing bowls for mixing ingredients, marinating, and storing prepped items.

6. **Measuring Cups and Spoons**:
Accurate measurements are crucial in
cooking. A set of measuring cups and
spoons is a must.

7. **Non-Stick Pans**: Non-stick pans
are great for sautéing, frying, and
cooking with less oil. They are easy to
clean as well.

8. **Saucepans and Pots**: Invest in a
range of sizes for boiling, simmering,
and preparing different dishes
simultaneously.

9. **Sheet Pan**: A large sheet pan is
useful for roasting vegetables, baking,
and preparing one-pan meals.

10. **Slow Cooker or Instant Pot**: These appliances are fantastic for set-it-and-forget-it cooking, making soups, stews, and tenderizing meats.

11. **Steamer Basket**: A steamer basket can help you steam vegetables, dumplings, and more without losing nutrients.

12. **Microplane Grater**: This tool is perfect for zesting citrus fruits, grating cheese, and adding finely grated spices.

13. **Tongs**: Tongs are versatile for flipping, tossing, and serving items while keeping your hands safe from heat.

14. **Whisk**: A whisk is essential for beating eggs, mixing sauces, and incorporating air into batters.

15. **Colander**: Use a colander for draining pasta, rinsing vegetables, and washing fruits.

16. **Peeler**: A vegetable peeler makes quick work of peeling fruits and vegetables.

17. **Oven Mitts or Pot Holders**: Safety is key, so have proper protection for handling hot pots and pans.

18. **Kitchen Timer**: A timer can help you manage multiple cooking tasks simultaneously and prevent overcooking.

19. **Storage Containers**: Have a variety of sizes for storing prepped ingredients and leftovers.

20. **Herb Stripper**: This handy tool helps you quickly remove leaves from herb stems.

21. **Can Opener**: If you use canned ingredients, a reliable can opener is a must.

Remember, the right tools can save you time and effort, making meal prep more enjoyable and efficient. Choose tools based on your cooking habits and preferences.

CHAPTER FOURTEEN

Sample Plant-Based Budget Meal

here's a sample plant-based budget meal plan for a day:

Breakfast:

Oatmeal with Banana and Almond Butter
-Rolled oats can be prepared with water or plant milk.
-Add a slice of banana and some almond butter on top.

Lunch:

Chickpea Salad Wrap
- Mash chickpeas with a fork and mix with diced vegetables (such as bell peppers, cucumbers, and tomatoes).
- Add a splash of lemon juice, a drizzle of olive oil, and season with salt and pepper.
In a whole wheat tortilla, enclose the ingredients.

Snack:

Carrot Sticks with Hummus

- Enjoy carrot sticks dipped in hummus for a crunchy and satisfying snack.

Dinner:

Lentil and Vegetable Stir-Fry
- Cook lentils and set aside.
- In a pan, stir-fry mixed vegetables (such as broccoli, bell peppers, and snap peas) with garlic and ginger.
- Add cooked lentils and a simple stir-fry sauce made from soy sauce, sesame oil, and a touch of maple syrup.
- Serve over brown rice or quinoa.

Dessert:

Mixed Berry Parfait
- Layer plant-based yogurt with mixed berries (such as strawberries, blueberries, and raspberries).
-Add some granola for crunch on top.
Remember to adjust portion sizes and ingredients based on your personal preferences and nutritional needs. This sample meal plan incorporates affordable plant-based staples like oats, lentils,chickpeas, vegetables,and fruits,which are all budget friendly option.

CHAPTER FIFTEEN

Frequently Asked Questions about Plant-Based Budget Meal Prep

Here are some frequently asked questions about plant-based budget meal prep:

1.is a plant-based diet more costly than the standard one?

Plant-based diets can be cost-effective, especially if you focus on whole foods like grains, legumes, fruits, and vegetables. These staples are often less expensive than animal products.

2. How can I save money while following a plant-based diet?

- Buy in bulk: Purchase items like beans, rice, oats, and grains in bulk to save money in the long run.
- Cook at home: Preparing meals from scratch is generally more affordable than buying pre-packaged foods.

- Shop seasonal produce: Choose fruits and vegetables that are in season, as they tend to be cheaper and fresher.
- Plan meals: Planning your meals for the week helps you buy only what you need and avoid unnecessary purchases.

3. What are some affordable sources of plant-based protein?

Legumes (beans, lentils, chickpeas), tofu, tempeh, quinoa, nuts, seeds, and whole grains like brown rice are excellent sources of affordable plant-based protein.

4. Are there budget-friendly alternatives to dairy products?

Yes, you can opt for plant-based milk alternatives like almond, soy, or oat milk. These can be cost-effective if you buy them in larger containers.

5. How can I prepare meals affordably?

- **Plan ahead**: Plan your meals for the week and create a shopping list based on what you need.

- **Batch cooking**:Prepare more food and save the leftovers for next meals.

- **Use frozen produce**: Frozen fruits and vegetables are often less expensive and retain their nutrients.

- **Repurpose leftovers**: Transform leftovers into new dishes to avoid waste.

6. Are there affordable options for plant-based snacks?

Yes, there are plenty of budget-friendly plant-based snacks:
- Fresh fruits and vegetables (carrot sticks, apple slices, etc.).
- Popcorn (air-popped without excessive butter or oil).

- Nuts and seeds (buy in bulk for cost savings).
- Homemade energy bars (made with oats, dried fruits, and nuts).

7. Can I get all the necessary nutrients on a budget-friendly plant-based diet?

Yes, you can. Focus on a variety of whole plant foods to ensure you're getting a balanced array of nutrients. Your meals should contain a variety of fruits, vegetables, whole grains, legumes, nuts, and seeds.

8. Are there affordable ways to add flavor to plant-based dishes?

Absolutely:
- Use herbs and spices for flavor without added cost.
- Make your own sauces and dressings at home using basic ingredients like vinegar, olive oil, lemon juice, and spices.
- Utilize condiments like mustard, hot sauce, and soy sauce to enhance flavor.

9. How can I make plant-based eating on a budget more exciting?

Experiment with different cuisines, flavors, and cooking techniques. Try new recipes, explore international dishes, and get creative with ingredient combinations to keep your meals interesting.

Remember, adopting a plant-based diet on a budget is about finding the balance between cost-effective staples and variety in your meals. With careful planning and smart shopping, you can enjoy delicious and nutritious plant-based meals without breaking the bank.

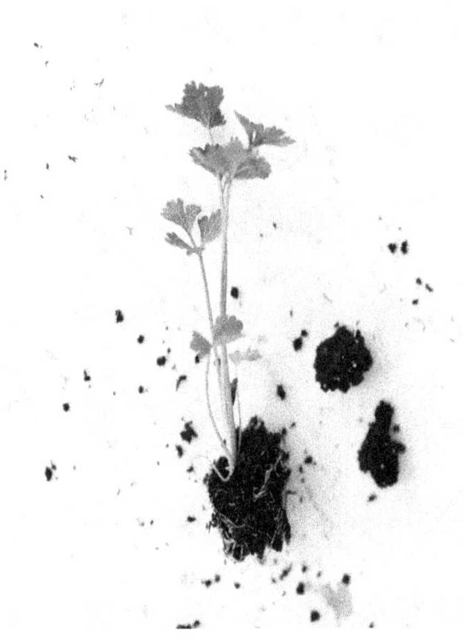

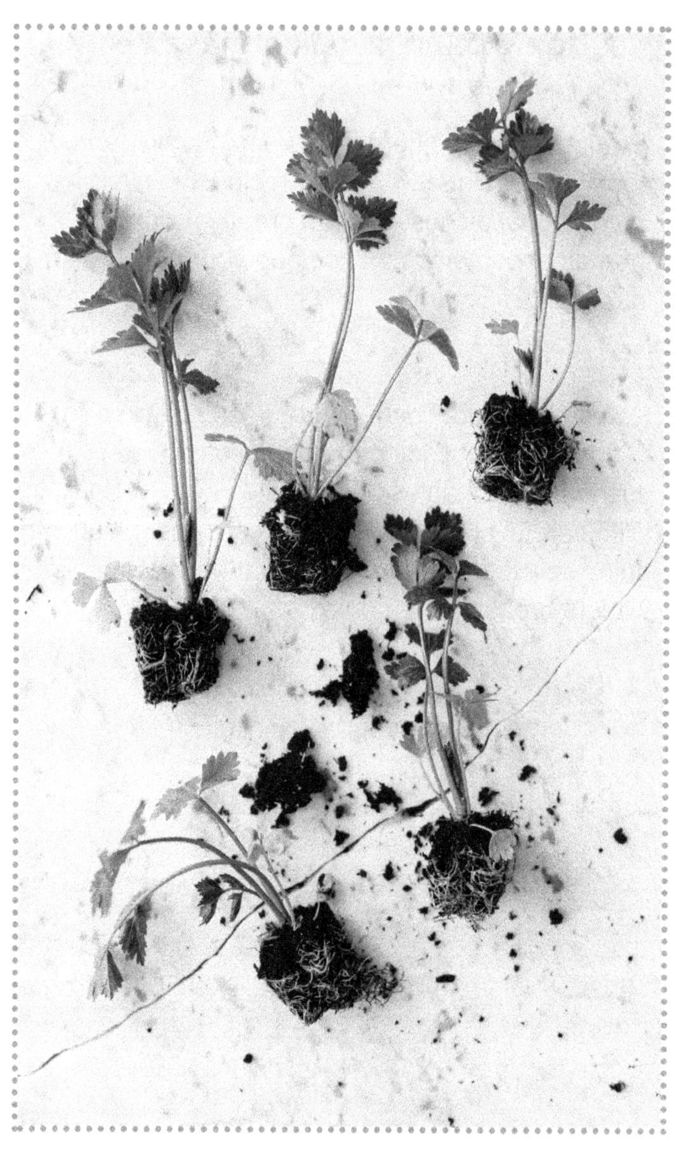

CHAPTER SIXTEEN

Embracing Sustainability in Your Plant-Based Journey

Embracing sustainability in your plant-based journey not only benefits your health but also contributes positively to the environment. Here are some ways to incorporate sustainability into your plant-based lifestyle:

1. Choose Local and Seasonal Foods:

Opt for locally grown and seasonal fruits and vegetables. This reduces the carbon footprint associated with transportation and supports local farmers.

2. Reduce Food Waste:

Plan your meals, store your food appropriately, and find inventive ways to use leftovers to reduce food waste.
Composting food scraps can also help divert waste from landfills.

3. Shop Mindfully:

Purchase items with minimal packaging and bring your own reusable bags and containers to reduce plastic waste.

4. Buy in Bulk:

Buying staples like grains, beans, nuts, and seeds in bulk reduces packaging waste and often costs less per unit.

5. Grow Your Own:

If possible, grow your own herbs, fruits, and vegetables at home. It's a rewarding way to decrease your reliance on store-bought produce.

6. Support Sustainable Brands:

Choose plant-based products from companies that prioritize sustainability, eco-friendly packaging, and ethical practices.

7. Reduce Energy Consumption:

Cook efficiently by using smaller appliances, such as microwaves and toaster ovens, which use less energy than ovens and stovetops.

8. Embrace Zero-Waste Cooking:

Use all parts of fruits and vegetables, including peels, stems, and tops. Make vegetable broths from scraps and explore creative ways to use every edible part.

9. Use Reusable Kitchen Tools:

Opt for reusable tools like cloth napkins, dish towels, and silicone baking mats instead of disposable paper products.

10. Avoid Single-Use Plastics:

Reduce your consumption of single-use plastics by using reusable water bottles, coffee cups, and food storage containers.

11. Support Plant-Based Agriculture:

Shift your support towards agricultural practices that are kinder to the environment, such as regenerative farming and organic practices.

12. Learn Preservation Techniques:

Explore methods like pickling, fermenting, and canning to extend the shelf life of produce and reduce waste.

13. Reduce Meat Substitutes:

While convenient, processed meat substitutes can have high environmental impacts due to processing. Focus on whole plant foods like legumes, grains, and vegetables.

14. Mindful Portion Control:

Cook and serve appropriate portion sizes to avoid overeating and minimize food waste.

15. Share and Educate:

Share your sustainable plant-based journey with friends and family. Encourage conversations about the positive environmental impacts of choosing plant-based options.

Remember, embracing sustainability in your plant-based journey involves making mindful choices that align with your values. Small changes can collectively lead to a significant reduction in your ecological footprint while enjoying a nutritious and compassionate diet.

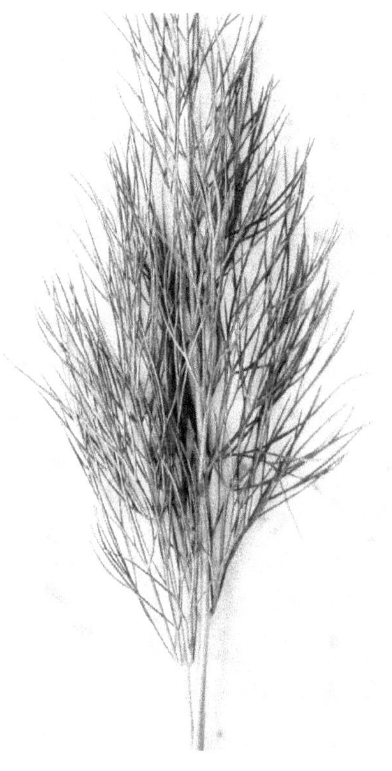

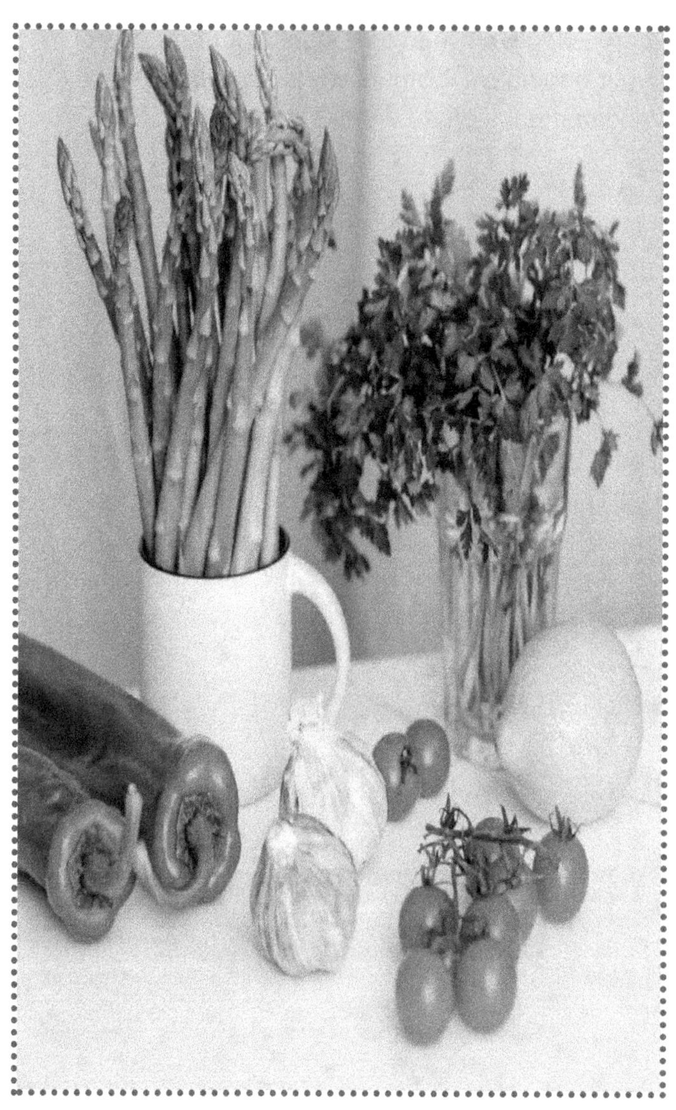

CHAPTER SEVENTEEN

Flavorful Spices and Sauces That Won't Break the Bank

Absolutely! Here are some flavorful spices and sauces that can add excitement to your dishes without straining your budget:

Spices:

1. **Cumin:** Adds a warm, earthy flavor to dishes like curries, soups, and roasted vegetables.

2. **Paprika:** Comes in various types (sweet, smoked, hot) and adds a rich, smoky flavor to stews, rice dishes, and grilled veggies.

3. **Turmeric:** Known for its bright color and earthy taste, it's great for curries, rice, and lentil dishes.

4. **Cinnamon:** Adds warmth and sweetness to both savory (like stews) and sweet (like oatmeal) dishes.

5. **Chili Powder:** Adds heat and depth to Mexican-inspired dishes, chili, and even roasted nuts.

6. **Garlic Powder:** Provides a convenient way to add garlic flavor to sauces, marinades, and roasted vegetables.

7. **Onion Powder:** Imparts a mild onion flavor to a variety of dishes, from sauces to stir-fries.

8. **Ginger:** Adds a zesty kick to stir-fries, curries, and marinades.

Sauces:

1. **Soy Sauce or Tamari:** Offers salty umami flavor to stir-fries, noodles, and marinades.

2. **Hot Sauce:** Adds a spicy kick to everything from tofu scrambles to soups.

3. **Salsa:** Versatile and budget-friendly, it's a flavorful addition to tacos, wraps, and salads.

4. **Hummus:** A creamy and tangy dip that works as a spread or sauce for sandwiches and wraps.

5. **Mustard:** Adds tanginess and depth to dressings, marinades, and sandwiches.

6.**Sauces:**
To personalize, add herbs and spices.
** Tomato sauce Paste:** The base for many sauces, from pasta to stews.

7. **Vinegar (Apple Cider, Balsamic, Rice):** Provides acidity to balance flavors in dressings, sauces, and roasted dishes.

8. **Tahini:** A sesame paste that adds richness and nuttiness to sauces, dressings, and dips.

9. **Lemon or Lime Juice:** Adds a burst of freshness to marinades, sauces, and grains.

Remember, a little goes a long way with spices and sauces. Experiment with combinations to find your favorite flavor profiles, and you'll be able to create delicious and budget-friendly meals with ease.

CHAPTER EIGHTEEN

Celebrating Special Occasions on a Budget

Celebrating special occasions on a budget can be just as memorable and meaningful. Here are some ideas to help you create wonderful moments without breaking the bank:

1. Homemade Gifts: Create personalized gifts, such as handmade crafts, baked goods, or a heartfelt letter. These show thought and effort.

2. Potluck Gathering: Invite friends and family for a potluck meal where everyone contributes a dish. It's a great way to share the celebration without bearing all the costs.

3. Outdoor Picnic: Plan a picnic at a local park or beach. Pack sandwiches, salads, and snacks for a budget-friendly and enjoyable day.

4. Movie Marathon: Have a movie or TV show marathon at home with close friends or family. Make popcorn, set up cozy blankets, and enjoy each other's company.

5. DIY Decorations: Create decorations using items you already have at home. Repurpose items, use paper crafts, or even make your own banners.

6. Game Night: Host a game night with board games, card games, or trivia. It's a fun and engaging way to celebrate without spending much.

7. Cooking Together: Prepare a special meal together with loved ones. This can be a fun and collaborative way to celebrate while also sharing the workload.

8. Nature Adventure: Go for a hike, nature walk, or visit a nearby beach or lake. Nature provides a beautiful backdrop for celebrating without costs.

9. Virtual Celebrations: If distance is a challenge, consider virtual celebrations. Host a video call with family and friends to celebrate together.

10. DIY Photo Booth: Create a DIY photo booth with props and a simple backdrop for fun and memorable photos.

11. Free Community Events: Check local event listings for free or low-cost community events happening on or around the occasion.

12. Memory Sharing: Ask friends and family to share their favorite memories or stories related to the occasion. This can be heartwarming and entertaining.

13. Write a Poem or Song: If you're creatively inclined, write a poem, song, or a short story to share with the celebrant.

14. Charitable Celebrations: Dedicate the occasion to a cause you care about. Instead of gifts, ask guests to make a donation to a chosen charity.

15. Spa Day at Home: **Treat** yourself or a loved one to a spa day at home with DIY facials, baths, and relaxation.

16. Cultural Potluck: Host a cultural potluck where guests bring dishes from different cuisines, allowing everyone to experience new flavors.

17. Scavenger Hunt: Organize a scavenger hunt with clues and hidden surprises for an exciting adventure.

Remember, the most important part of celebrating is spending quality time with loved ones and creating cherished memories. With a little creativity and thoughtfulness, you can make special occasions memorable without straining your budget.

CHAPTER NINETEEN

Plant-Based Meal Prep Success Stories

Certainly! Here are a few plant-based meal prep success stories that showcase the positive impact of adopting a plant-based lifestyle:

1. Increased Energy and Weight Loss:

Sarah, a busy working professional, struggled with fatigue and excess weight. After transitioning to a plant-based diet and committing to meal prepping, she experienced a significant increase in energy levels. She lost weight gradually over time and felt more confident and motivated to stay active.

2. Improved Digestion and Gut Health:

John had struggled with digestive issues for years. After switching to a plant-based diet and focusing on whole, fiber-rich foods, his digestion improved significantly. He found relief from bloating and discomfort and noticed better gut health overall.

3. Budget-Friendly Transformation:

Emily, a college student on a tight budget, decided to explore a plant-based diet to save money on groceries. She discovered that beans, lentils, rice, and seasonal produce were not only affordable but also nutritious. Through careful meal planning and batch cooking, Emily successfully navigated her college years on a budget while nourishing her body with plant-based meals.

4. Athletic Performance Boost:

Mark, a fitness enthusiast, was initially concerned that a plant-based diet wouldn't provide enough protein for his active lifestyle. However, he discovered that incorporating beans, tofu, tempeh, and whole grains into his diet provided ample protein. Not only did he maintain his muscle mass, but he also experienced improved endurance during workouts.

5. Reversing Chronic Health Conditions:

Linda was diagnosed with high blood pressure and high cholesterol. Her doctor recommended adopting a plant-based diet to help manage these conditions. After committing to the lifestyle change and preparing plant-based meals at home, Linda's blood pressure and cholesterol levels improved, reducing her reliance on medications.

6. Family Bonding and Healthier Choices:

The Johnson family decided to transition to a plant-based diet as a family. They found that meal prepping together on weekends not only saved time during busy weekdays but also strengthened their family bond. Their children became more adventurous eaters and developed a taste for diverse plant-based foods.

These success stories highlight how plant-based meal prep can lead to a wide range of positive outcomes, from increased energy and weight loss to improved digestion and better overall health. While individual experiences may vary, many people find that adopting a plant-based lifestyle and incorporating meal prepping strategies positively impact their physical and emotional well-being.

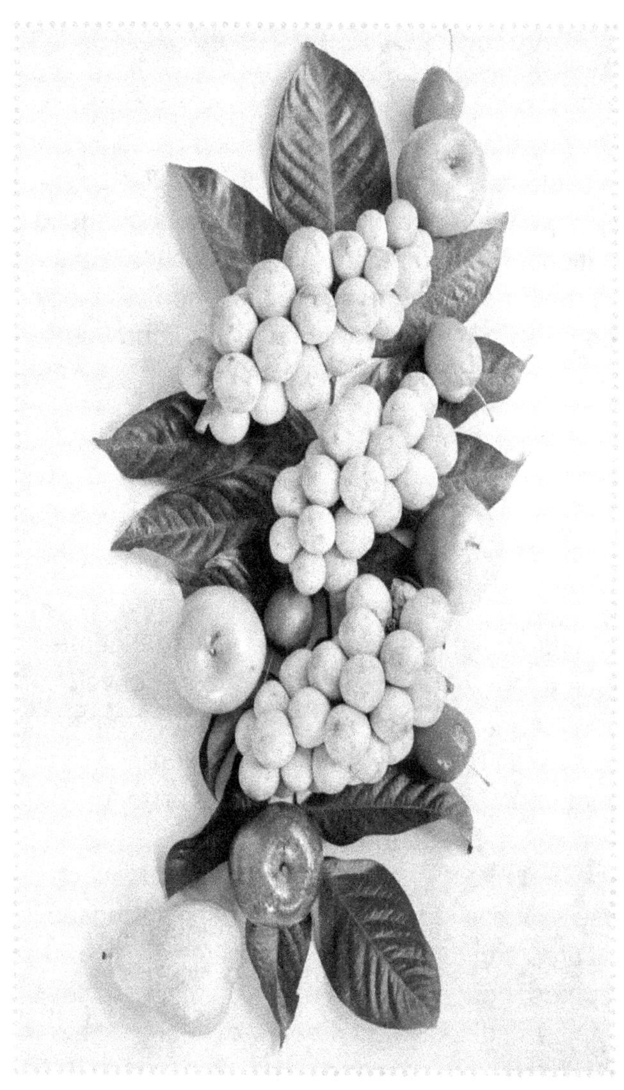

CONCLUSION

Nourishing Your Body and Wallet Through Plant-Based Eating

Embracing a plant-based diet while on a budget offers a multitude of benefits that extend beyond just your wallet. Here are some compelling advantages to consider.

1. Healthier Lifestyle: Plant-based diets are rich in vitamins, minerals, and fiber, which can contribute to better overall health. They're associated with lower risk of chronic diseases like heart disease, diabetes, and certain cancers.

2. Eco-Friendly Impact: By choosing plant-based foods, you're reducing the demand for animal agriculture, which is a major contributor to greenhouse gas emissions, deforestation, and water usage.

3. Culinary Creativity: Plant-based eating encourages you to explore new flavors, ingredients, and cooking methods. This can lead to greater culinary creativity and a more diverse palate.

4. Sustainable Eating Habits: Learning to prioritize seasonal and local produce, minimize food waste, and prepare meals at home fosters sustainable eating habits that benefit both your health and the planet.

5. Budget Freedom: Plant-based eating can be cost-effective, freeing up funds for other priorities in your life. With smart shopping, meal planning, and batch cooking, you can stretch your budget without compromising nutrition.

6. Ethical Considerations: By choosing plant-based options, you're making a compassionate choice for animals and supporting ethical food practices.

7. Positive Community Impact: Sharing your plant-based journey with friends and family can inspire others to make more sustainable and health-conscious choices.

Incorporating plant-based meals into your routine doesn't have to be overwhelming. Start small, experiment with new ingredients and recipes, and gradually build a collection of go-to meals that work for your tastes and budget. With thoughtful

planning, you can nourish your body, your wallet,
and the planet through plant-based eating.

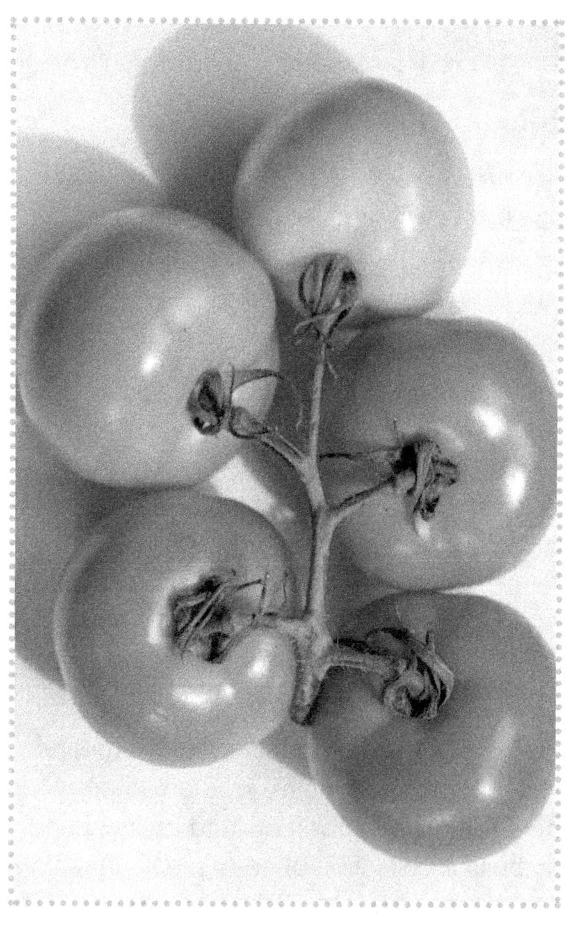

DAILY MEAL REMARKS

Day	Recipe	Remark